DASH Diet

6-Week DASH Diet Plan for Beginners for a Faster Weight Loss, Fitness and More Energy

By Jennifer DeMoines

Table of Contents

Chapter 1: What is the DASH diet?

DASH stands for Dietary Approaches to Stop Hypertension. Unlike many fad diets that became popular over the last years, DASH diet is based on the recent scientific research conducted by the National Institute of Health and is recommended by the United States Department of Agriculture (USDA) as one of the best ways to maintain a healthy lifestyle, lower blood pressure, decrease risk of cancer, stroke and heart disease. While the DASH diet was not originally designed with the specific goal of weight loss, weight loss is a frequent and desired side-effect of following the DASH approach.

The DASH diet focuses on limiting consumption of foods containing high levels of sodium and fat, while, at the same time, encouraging consumption of fruits, vegetables, whole grains and lean meats. What differentiates the DASH diet from many others (and what many find appealing) is that there are no foods that are specifically banned by the program (think red meats, sweets, alcohol or caffeine). In addition, no strict calorie-counting or food weighing is required. Instead, the DASH diet encourages "everything in moderation" approach, where foods that are higher in sodium, fat or sugar are allowed in small amounts.

What are the foods recommended by the DASH diet?

The following chart outlines different food groups and daily amounts recommended by the DASH diet.

Food group	Servings per day	Examples
Whole grains	7-8	Whole-wheat bread, cereal, brown rice, whole-wheat pasta
Fruits	4-5	Apples, bananas, peaches, pears, plums, apricots
Vegetables	5-6	Tomatoes, potatoes, carrots, beets, broccoli, asparagus
Lean meats	2-3	Poultry, fish, seafood
Dairy	2-3	Low fat milk, yogurt, cheese
Healthy fats	5-6	Nuts, seeds, peanut butter

The above foods are rich in fiber, vitamins, minerals, proteins and all the nutrients needed to maintain a healthy lifestyle. At the same time, the DASH diet recommends one limits their consumption of foods that raise blood pressure or create insulin spikes, even if temporarily. These include red and processed meats (beef, lamb, sausage, and lunch meats), alcohol, caffeinated beverages, and sweets.

What should I use as a serving?

One of the questions that you may ask is what exactly constitutes one serving. The following table provides a guide to what the weight and size of 1 serving is in each of the food groups.

Food group	Size of one serving
Whole grains	1 slice of bread, 1/2 cup of cooked cereal, rice or pasta (size of a 1/2 baseball).
Fruits	1 medium fruit (size of a baseball); 1/2 cup chopped, cooked or canned fruit
Vegetables	1 cup (size of a small fist)
Lean meats	2 to 3 ounces of cooked lean meat, poultry or fish
Dairy	1 cup of milk or yogurt, 1 1/2 ounces of cheese.

What if I don't like an entire food group?

A common question is what to do if you do not like a particular type of food or are not too fond of a particular nutrition group. Good news – DASH Diet does allow you to have the freedom of choice of what you eat, and only suggest placing more emphasis on some foods and reducing others.

- **Use spices**. Most of us have some spices at the back of the kitchen cabinets, tucked away for a long time, waiting for their prime time. To avoid all the foods tasting plain and bland, bring out those spices. Without the addition of salts and trans fats, you can still make your food stand out and have texture and rich flavor – all at a healthy pace.

- **Try a new dish.** Select a new dish from the food group that you have not tried before. Most restaurants will have something you did not try before, labeled with a heart icon or similar. Those are usually specifically prepared with heart- and blood-pressure mind and do taste great. Give 'em a chance!

- **Include small amount in a recipe in another dish.** For example, if you do not like vegetables, cook some pasta and add peas to it.

- **Try again later.** Even if you don't like a certain food at first, try it again in a few weeks. Your taste buds will adapt to the new healthy lifestyle, and you may love the same food later.

Chapter 2: How do I get started?

Before we get started on your journey to a healthier new you, let's review some important strategies to keep in mind throughout the process:

1. **Ease into the plan.** Very few of those who decide to change something suddenly or quit cold turkey succeed long-term. The trick is to make the change gradually. If today, the only vegetables in your diet include an occasional slice of tomato on top of your hamburger, do not think that you can suddenly start eating the entire recommended 7-8 servings of vegetables every day and stick to this new habit. A much more sensible approach would be to start adding 1-2 servings of vegetables to your diet every couple of weeks.

2. **Define success and set specific, measurable goals.** To succeed at anything, you first need to define what success means to you and determine how you will measure it. Set some goals, but make sure that these are measurable, achievable and have a specific timeline. If weight loss is your goal, set your target weight and the date by which you want to hit that goal. Keep in mind, that on average, it is not healthy or realistic to lose more than 2 pounds of weight per week. In addition, if the date by which you've determined you will achieve your goal is more than 1-2 months into the future, you have to set sub-goals for shorter time periods to keep yourself from being discouraged.

3. **Introduce a *calorie deficit*.** For the first week, try keeping you portions to 1,900 calories a day. If weight loss is among your goals, in addition to reducing the blood pressure, the following week, try further widening this deficit by going for 1,800 calorie totals. Write down your calorie consumption across all meals, plus snacks, each day. If you are tech savvy, use your favorite app, like Google Fit, to measure your fitness progress or track your calorie account.

4. **Reward yourself.** Very simply, you need to celebrate even small successes to keep yourself on track to reach your target goals. That is, every time you reach a milestone, treat yourself to something you enjoy (and I do not mean food), try a new experience, like buy yourself a dress when you reach a certain size, go scuba dive, book a quick weekend getaway, etc.

5. **Don't punish yourself.** Even if you slip up, do not make a big deal out of it. Stay busy. Being occupied with activities away from the dining table can help you keep your mind away from the foods you may still be craving.

6. **Cut sodium in other ways.** Use spices or flavorings instead of salt. Rinse canned foods to remove some of the sodium. Check food labels to buy foods that are low in sodium content. If you still want a snack, choose foods that have low calorie count but come in a high volume. For example, popcorn works well for that purpose.

7. **Don't forget to exercise.** Exercise is known to lower blood pressure. It will let you achieve the results even faster by burning more calories, increasing your metabolism, producing endorphins that keep you from emotional stress-eating. Additionally, it builds muscle to make you look fit, trains heart and has many other long-term health benefits.

In general, try to dedicate at least 10 minutes to light exercise every morning before breakfast, and spend about 30 minutes at least three times a week doing moderate to high energy activity, like power walking or light jogging. The best activity is something that you can do outdoors. Remember to stick to your exercise routine and complete the activities you planned regardless of the weather.

8. **Enlist a friend.** Friend will keep you accountable and help you stick to the plan. You can organize an informal healthy competition between each other, which will make exercising more fun – it will not be just about running on the treadmill. Share and exchange meal plans with your friend. I often find that you can build on each other's program and encourage results.

9. **Don't give up.** It is critical to stick with it, regardless of the short term results. The results won't come immediately and vary drastically depending on individual metabolism, though DASH Diet is known to bring results in as little as 14 days. If weight gain is a

priority for you, you may find yourself hitting a plateau. Don't despair – the results will come. If you give up too soon, you may not only lose the results you already achieved, but may actually regress beyond the starting point!

Chapter 3: Week-by-week plan

Week 1: Let's focus on adding fruits and vegetables

The most fun way to start DASH diet is with a trip to a grocery store to stock up on food! That's right – we want to buy more food! Though this time, we are not going to the store for the foods with any trans fats or cholesterol. Instead, we're on the lookout for the healthy fruits and veggies. Go ahead, splurge on what's fun! Raspberries or apricots may cost more outside of the season, but will make a good snack that replaces foods that are high in saturated fats. Does your store carry tangy grapefruits? How about papaya? When was the last time you tried mangos?

Nuts are highly recommended during DASH Diets as well. If you decide to buy a pack of nuts, go for the unsalted, unroasted kind – the raw nuts. They will keep you feeling full longer, and they are easy to pack into a purse or a bag and carry with you.

For the exercise, we want to slowly ease into a light to moderate exercise routing. Daily routine that keep you active is better than one burst of exercise every week.

Week 2: Let's go after potassium, calcium and magnesium

Three critical chemicals in your body, namely, potassium, calcium and magnesium, come from a variety of sources. Food that are high in potassium include avocados, mushrooms, beans and most leafy greens. Yogurt, fish and bananas can also typically provide a good supply of potassium.

For calcium, again choose leafy greens, dairy, broccoli, and beans. Almonds are a great source as well. You will find the most magnesium in most nuts, seeds, fish, beans, avocados, and – again – in the same leafy greens.

Try starting a meal – any meal – with an apple or another fruit, plus a glass of fresh water. This step will achieve two goals: first, fruits rich in fiber will generally keep you feeling full longer, resulting in fewer cravings. A glass of water will fool your stomach into perceiving the extra weight and volume as food. Those two tricks will help you eat less by the end of the meal.

During this second week, it is critical to reduce consumption of butter and fats from dairy, like cream. If you've ever wanted to try being vegetarian for a week, now is the perfect time. Try putting off the red meats for a few days. You may actually feel more energy.

Week 3: Let's gradually reduce sodium

Most people who start with the DASH Diet typically start with an "Average American diet," as defined by the National Heart, Lung and Blood Institute (NHLBI), which contains roughly 3,000 mg of sodium per day. This week, we will perform the first reduction in sodium down to 2,400 mg, which is typically considered an intermediate sodium intake level by the dietitians. Do not slash the sodium entirely all at once from your diet: you do not want to go too abruptly to avoid cravings.

By this third week, you should start feeling the initial results, and the doctor may confirm the successful progress: according to The American Heart Association (AHA), by the end of this week, the blood pressure monitor readings should be able to reflect the results of DASH Dieting. By now, your cholesterol is likely to start improving.

Week 4: Let's focus on healthy fluids!

To succeed in DASH Diet, NIH (National Institutes of Health) under the US Department of Health, that performed the trials that measured impact of the DASH Diet on the long-term health of the patients, recommends limiting sweetened beverages and sweets. They also recommend reducing the intake of alcohol. Replace that glass of wine with a glass of fresh water. If you want, use some ice. Add a wedge of fresh lemon (and squeeze it!) to give you water some flavor and body.

Instead of the coffee, try decaf. Try to limit the amount of meals you eat while going out. Try to cut snacks and restaurant foods, especially those heavy on the salt, like chips or burgers. This should help us further slash the sodium consumption down to 1,500 mg per day – a healthy level.

Finally, try fruits that are high on water content. Watermelons, melons, cantaloupes are all a fair game, plus they taste great!

Don't forget to exercise.

Week 5: Let's keep up the healthy activity and moderate exercise!

By now, you will definitely be feeling the effect of the DASH Diet. Your blood pressure likely improved: systolic pressure should have dropped by at least 6 mm Hg, and diastolic – by 3mm Hg. If you started the diet with hypertension, you will likely see 11 and 6 mm Hg decrease on average, according to NIH.

Find opportunities to exercise outdoors. Walk in the park, take the stairs at work, and get a standing desk at work if you can. Many people choose to buy FitBit or a pedometer to keep themselves motivated. If you are doing 10,000 steps a day, you're doing great!

Moderate exercise should help you sustain the effect.

Week 6: Let's make this a habit!

Focus on making the lifestyle a habit. This final week, do not worry about changing your diet. Our goal is to turn the progress from the past five weeks a regular habit that is easy to maintain in the day-to-day activities. Maintain the same levels of sodium and light caffeine intake as a week before, but do not sweat over your diet charts as closely as you did in the recent weeks.

By now, you are likely experiencing a higher level of alertness, are feeling refreshed, and your mood has likely generally improved. Enjoy your new inflow of energy, better sleep, and in general a sense of better well-being!

Chapter 4: 5 Day Sample Menu

The following is a 5-day sample menu followed by the recipes* of some of the lunch and dinner entrees specified below.

Day 1

Breakfast	Lunch	Dinner
• 2 egg whites omelet with tomatoes, onions, green peppers, low-fat cheese • 1 cup of fresh fruits • Herbal tea	• Tuna sandwich made with 2 slices of whole-wheat bread, avocado, 3 ounces of canned tuna, 2 tablespoons light mayonnaise, lettuce, tomato • 1 serving of Apple-Fennel Slaw • 1 cup fat-free milk	• 1 serving of Baked Salmon with Asian Marinade* • 1 cup cooked whole-wheat rice, no added salt • 2 cups mixed salad greens with • 1 tablespoon of olive oil • 1 apple • Sparkling water

Day 2

Breakfast	Lunch	Dinner
• 1 serving of cereal • 1 banana • 1 cup fat-free milk	• 1 serving of Citrus salad* • 1 slice whole-wheat toast • ½ cup of raw sliced bell peppers • Water	• 1 serving of Balsamic Roast Chicken* • 1 cup mashed potatoes, no added salt • 2 cups of asparagus cooked with spices and 1 tablespoon of olive oil • 1 cup of fresh fruit • Herbal tea

Day 3

Breakfast	Lunch	Dinner
• 1 slice whole-wheat toast • 1 teaspoon of trans-fat free margarine • 1 yogurt • 1 cup of grapes • Herbal tea	• 1 whole-wheat pita with chopped chicken, fresh vegetables and low-fat cheese • 1 serving of Blue Cheese, Spinach, and Walnut Salad* • 1 cup fat-free milk	• 1 serving of Beef Stew* • 1 nectarine • Sparkling water

Day 4

Breakfast	Lunch	Dinner
• 1 whole-wheat bagel with 2 tablespoons peanut butter (no salt added) • 1 medium orange • Decaffeinated coffee	• Tuna sandwich made with 2 slices of whole-wheat bread, avocado, 3 ounces of canned tuna, 2 tablespoons light mayonnaise, lettuce, tomato • ½ cup of raw baby carrots • 1 cup fat-free milk	• 1 serving of Broiled Scallops with Sweet Lime Sauce* • 1 cup cooked risotto, no added salt • 1 cup chopped tomatoes and cucumbers • 1 tablespoon of olive oil • 1 cup of mixed fruit • Herbal tea

Day 5

Breakfast	Lunch	Dinner
<ul><li>1 cup of oatmeal</li><li>1 yogurt</li><li>1 medium apple</li><li>1 cup fat-free milk</li></ul>	<ul><li>1 serving of Greek salad*</li><li>1 beef or lamp kebab</li><li>1 sliced pear</li><li>1 cup fat-free milk</li></ul>	<ul><li>1 serving of Curried Pork Tenderloin with Apple Cider*</li><li>1 serving of Potato salad*</li><li>2 cups cooked vegetables</li><li>1 peach</li><li>Sparkling water</li></ul>

Chapter 5: Sample Recipes

Greek Salad

Serving Size: 1 Cup

Servings: 8

Ingredients

- 1 Tbsp. Red Wine Vinegar

- 1 Tbsp. Lemon Juice

- 2 tsp. Fresh Oregano, Chopped

- ½ tsp. Salt

- ¼ tsp. Pepper

- 2 ½ Tbsp. Extra-Virgin Olive Oil

- 1 Eggplant, 1 ½ lbs.

- 1 lb. Spinach

- 1 Hothouse Cucumber

- 1 Tomato

- ½ Onion

- 2 Tbsp. Greek Olives, Pitted, and Chopped

- 2 Tbsp. Crumbled Feta Cheese

Directions

1. Prepare the eggplant by chopping off the ends, peeling it, and dicing it into one inch pieces. Prepare the spinach by rinsing it and cutting off the stems. Prepare the cucumber by slicing it.

2. Place a rack in your oven on the lower third of the oven and preheat your oven to 450° Fahrenheit. Coat a baking sheet with some olive oil cooking spray.

3. Whisk together the vinegar through the pepper in a small bowl to make the dressing. Add the olive oil in slowly to emulsify it. Refrigerate until you're ready for it.

4. Place the eggplant on the baking sheet and spray it with some olive oil cooking spray. Roast the eggplant for ten minutes and turn the cubes, then roast another eight to ten minutes. Allow them to cool completely.

5. Combine the remainder of the ingredients and the eggplant in a bowl. Toss generously and then add the vinaigrette and serve.

Citrus Salad

Serves: 4

Ingredients

- 1 Grapefruit

- 2 Oranges

- 2 Tbsp. Orange Juice

- 2 Tbsp. Olive Oil

- 1 Tbsp. Balsamic Vinegar

- Sweetener

- 4 C. Spring Greens

- 2 Tbsp. Pine Nuts

Directions

1. Peel away the skin of the orange and the pith. Then gently free the fruit from the membrane by slicing it down the middle and squeezing gently. Repeat the same process with the grapefruit.

2. Whisk the orange juice, vinegar and olive oil together in a bowl and add the sweetener to your preference. Then pour it over the fruit segments and toss them gently to combine.

3. Divide your greens amongst plates or bowl and top with the fruit and the dressing mixture. Then add about a half a tablespoon of pine nuts to the top and serve immediately.

Blue Cheese, Spinach, and Walnut Salad

Serves: 12

Serving Size: 2 Cups

Ingredients

- 4 tsp. Olive Oil

- 2 Tbsp. Balsamic Vinegar

- 1 Tbsp. Maple Syrup

- ¼ tsp. Nutmeg

- 3 tsp. Low-Fat Yogurt, Plain

- 2 lbs. Spinach

- ½ C. Red Onion, Sliced

- 1 ½ C. Cucumbers, Sliced

- 1 ½ C. Grape Tomatoes

- ¼ C. Chopped Walnuts

- ¼ C. Blue Cheese, Crumbled

Directions

1. Combine all of the ingredients for the dressing in a food processor, the olive oil through the yogurt, and then chill.

2. Combine the spinach with the dressing and place a generous cup onto plates.

3. Layer the vegetables on top with the walnuts and blue cheese to garnish.

Serves: 4

Ingredients

- 1 Fennel Bulb, Sliced Thinly

- 1 Granny Smith Apple, Sliced Thinly

- 2 Carrots, Grated

- 2 Tbsp. Raisins

- 1 Tbsp. Olive Oil

- 1 tsp. Sugar

- ½ C. Apple Juice

- 2 Tbsp. Apple Cider Vinegar

- 4 Lettuce Leaves

Directions

1. Combine the first four ingredients in a bowl to make your slaw. Then drizzle it with the olive oil and cover it to put it in the refrigerator.

2. In a saucepan, place in the sugar and apple juice. Cook over medium heat until it's reduced to about a quarter of a cup or around ten minutes. Remove it from the heat and cool before adding in the cider vinegar. Then pour that over the slaw and stir to combine well.

3. Chill in the refrigerator before serving over a lettuce leaf.

Potato Salad

Servings: 8

Serving Size: ¾ C.

Ingredients

- 1 lb. Potatoes, Boiled and Diced

- 1 Onion, Minced

- 1 Carrot, Diced

- 2 Celery Ribs, Diced

- 2 Tbsp. Dill, Minced

- 1 tsp. Pepper

- ¼ C. Low-Fat Mayonnaise

- 1 Tbsp. Dijon Mustard

- 2 Tbsp. Red Wine Vinegar

Directions

1. Place the pepper through the red wine vinegar in a bowl and mix thoroughly.

2. Then add in the remainder of the ingredients and incorporate well.

3. You can choose to serve chilled or serve hot.

Baked Salmon with Asian Marinade

Serves: 2

Serving Size: 1 Filet

Ingredients

- ½ C. Pineapple Juice

- 2 Cloves Garlic, Minced

- 1 tsp. Low-Sodium Soy Sauce

- ¼ tsp. Ground Ginger

- 2 Salmond Fillets

- ¼ tsp. Sesame Oil

- Pepper to Taste

- 1 C. Fresh Fruit (Pineapple, Papaya, or Mango)

Directions

1. Add the pineapple juice through the ginger to a bowl and incorporate well.

2. Arrange the salmon in a baking dish and pour the mixture over top. Marinate in the refrigerator for one hour and turn the salmon every fifteen minutes.

3. Preheat your oven to 375° Fahrenheit and coat two pieces of aluminum foil with some cooking spray.

4. Place the salmon on the aluminum foil and drizzle with the sesame oil. Sprinkle each with the pepper and ½ a cup of diced fruit.

5. Wrap the foil around the salmon and seal well. Then bake until it's opaque, about ten minutes on either side.

Balsamic Roast Chicken

Serves: 8

Serving Size: 1/8 Recipe

Ingredients

- 1 Chicken, About 4 lbs.

- 1 Tbsp. Rosemary

- 1 Garlic Clove

- 1 Tbsp. Olive Oil

- 1/8 tsp. Pepper

- 8 Sprigs Rosemary

- ½ C. Balsamic Vinegar

- 1 tsp. Brown Sugar

Directions

1. Preheat your oven to 350° Fahrenheit.

2. Mince the rosemary and garlic and combine in a bowl. Loosen the skin from the skin and rub it with olive oil and the herb mixture. Sprinkle with some black pepper and place to rosemary sprigs in the chicken's cavity. Truss your chicken.

3. Place it in a roasting pan and roast for twenty minutes per pound, about an hour and twenty minutes. Baste every fifteen minutes with the pan juices.

4. Combine the balsamic vinegar and brown sugar in a saucepan and heat until it's warmed and the sugar dissolves. Be sure not to boil it!

5. Carve the chicken, remove the skin, and top with the vinegar mixture. Garnish with the rosemary sprigs that remain and serve.

Beef Stew

Serves: 4

Serving Size: 2 C.

Ingredients

- 1 lb. Beef Steak

- 2 tsp. Canola Oil

- 2 C. Onion, Diced

- 1 C. Celery, Diced

- 1 C. Roma Tomatoes, Diced

- ½ C. Sweet Potato, Diced

- ½ C. White Potato with Skin, Diced

- ½ C. Mushrooms, Diced

- 1 C. Carrot, Diced

- 4 Garlic Cloves, Chopped

- 1 C. Kale, Chopped

- ¼ C. Barley

- ¼ C. Red Wine Vinegar

- 1 tsp. Balsamic Vinegar

- 3 C. Low-Sodium Beef or Vegetable Stock

- 1 tsp. Sage

- 1 tsp. Thyme, Minced

- 1 Tbsp. Parsley, Minced

- 1 Tbsp. Oregano, Dried

- 1 tsp. Dried Rosemary

- Pepper to Taste

Directions

1. Preheat a grill or the broiler and cook the steak for twelve minutes, turning once. Remove from the heat and prepare the vegetables.

2. Saute the vegetables in a stock pot over medium-high heat until they're slightly brown, around ten minutes. Then add in the barley and cook another five minutes.

3. Pat the meat dry with a paper towel and dice it into half inch pieces. Add it to the pot and add the remainder of the ingredients. Cook for one hour.

Broiled Scallops with Sweet Lime Sauce

Serves: 4

Serving Size: ¼ Recipe

Ingredients

- 4 Tbsp. Honey

- 2 Tbsp. Lime Juice

- 1 Tbsp. Olive Oil

- 1 lb. Sea Scallops, Rinsed and Patted Dry

- 2 tsp. Lime Peel, Grated

- 1 Lime, Sliced into Four Wedges

Directions

1. Preheat your broiler and place the rack four inches from the top. Cover a baking sheet with aluminum foil and spray generously with the cooking spray.

2. Whisk the honey, oil, and lime juice together in a bowl and add the scallops. Toss to coat.

3. Arrange them on the baking sheet and broil about five minutes. Turn them over and broil another minute to get the other side golden.

4. Divide them onto four plates and pour any juices on the baking sheet over them. Sprinkle with the lime peel and serve with a lime wedge.

Curried Pork Tenderloin with Apple Cider

Serves: 6

Serving Size: 3 oz.

Ingredients

- 16 oz. Pork Tenderloin, Sliced into Six Pieces

- 1 ½ Tbsp. Curry Powder

- 1 Tbsp. Extra-Virgin Olive Oil

- 2 Onions, Chopped

- 2 C. Apple Cider, Divided

- 1 Apple, Seeded, Peeled, and Chopped

- 1 Tbsp. Cornstarch

Directions

1. Season your pork with the curry powder and allow it to rest for fifteen minutes.

2. Meanwhile, in a skillet, heat the oil. When it's ready, add the pork and turn it once, browning on both sides for a total of five to ten minutes. Remove from the skillet and set aside.

3. Add the onions and sauté them until they're soft and golden. Add in one and a half cups of the apple cider and reduce the heat until it's a simmer. Simmer until it's half its original volume.

4. Add the apple, cornstarch and the remainder of the apple cider to the pan. Then stir and cook about two minutes. Return the pork to the skillet and simmer another five minutes.

5. Pour the thickened sauce over the meat on a serving platter and serve.

Chapter 6: Results you should expect from the DASH Diet

You should expect a number of positive changes in your life that you experience and feel thanks to the DASH Diet. Among the top benefits are the following three things.

Result 1: Lower blood pressure

Due to the lower consumption of sodium, and higher consumption of healthy fiber and lean protein, along with a higher amount of magnesium, calcium and potassium in your diet, your blood pressure should drop noticeably, and your doctor is likely to see a meaningful difference in your "before" and "after" numbers. Additionally, though the DASH Diet, you have likely lowered your LDL cholesterol – the bad type of cholesterol. Both of these factors (lower blood pressure and lower LDL) are associated with the cardiovascular disease – so decrease in both is a good thing.

Result 2: Better mood

Your liver has to deal with fewer spikes of sugar in your blood, especially if you added a regular level of moderate exercise to your diet. You feel more energetic and have fewer high/low energy fluctuations.

Result 3: Reduced risk of stroke or heart problems

According to the US News and World Report, DASH Diet was named #1 for the Best Diet Overall. If you chose to stick to the plan above, you are on the right path towards a better health. Keep in mind that you need to keep up the diet - DASH Diet only works when you keep up with your long-term plan and goals. Buy yourself a good fitness monitor and monitor your progress daily.

The easiest way to slip is by not paying attention at your food choices while eating out. Salty foods or foods full of saturated fats may feel great short term, but will make sticking to the diet much harder long-term. Also, remember to drink alcohol in moderation!

Chapter 7: Conclusion

The DASH diet is all about lowering your blood pressure and reducing hypertension through gradually moving to a healthier life-style. The DASH diet does not offer a fast weight loss solution, but, instead, focuses on helping you form healthier eating habits and keeping you from going to the extremes by offering plenty of variety.

I hope you enjoyed this book on the DASH diet.

Thank You!

Jennifer DeMoines

Printed in Great Britain
by Amazon